THE USE OF ERYTHROMYCIN.

The Ultimate Guide to Treating Bacteria infections and The Alternative Approaches to Antibiotic resistance Therapy

Lila Evergreen

Disclaimer

This document provides general information about erythromycin, an antibiotic medication. It is not intended to be a substitute for professional medical advice, diagnosis, or treatment. Always seek the advice of your physician or other qualified health provider with any questions you may have regarding a medical condition.

CHAPTER ONE

Introduction to Erythromycin:

Erythromycin is a broad-spectrum antibiotic belonging to the macrolide class. Discovered in the early 1950s, it has been widely used in clinical practice for decades. The medication is derived from the soil bacterium *Streptomyces erythraeus*.

Historical Context:

- First introduced in the 1950s.
- Initially isolated from a soil sample in the Philippines.
- Considered one of the first macrolide antibiotics.

Chemical Structure:

- A large lactone ring with neutral and acidic sugars attached.

- Structurally related to other macrolide antibiotics like azithromycin and clarithromycin.

Mode of Action:

- Inhibits bacterial protein synthesis by binding to the 50S subunit of the bacterial ribosome.
- Prevents the translocation step of protein synthesis.
- Effective against a broad spectrum of bacteria, both Gram-positive and some Gram-negative.

Forms and Administration:

- Available in various formulations, including oral tablets, capsules, and intravenous solutions.
- Dosage forms may vary based on the indication and patient characteristics.

Indications:

- Used to treat respiratory tract infections, skin and soft tissue infections, and some sexually transmitted infections.
- Sometimes prescribed as a prophylactic antibiotic in certain situations.

Pharmacokinetics:

- Absorption may be influenced by food.
- Metabolized in the liver and excreted primarily in the bile.

Resistance Issues:

- Resistance to erythromycin has been observed, limiting its efficacy in some cases.
- Cross-resistance with other macrolides may occur.

Current Usage and Importance:

- Despite the emergence of newer antibiotics, erythromycin continues to be an essential part of the antibiotic armamentarium.
- It may be a preferred choice in specific clinical scenarios or when alternative antibiotics are contraindicated.

Conclusion:

- Erythromycin remains a vital antibiotic with a rich history and diverse applications in the treatment of bacterial infections. Understanding its mode of action, indications, and limitations is crucial for healthcare professionals to ensure its optimal and responsible use.

CHAPTER TWO

Mechanism of Action of Erythromycin:

Erythromycin, a macrolide antibiotic, exerts its antimicrobial effects by interfering with bacterial protein synthesis. The primary target of erythromycin is the bacterial ribosome, specifically the 50S subunit. The mechanism of action can be broken down into several key steps:

1. Binding to the Ribosome:

- Erythromycin binds reversibly to the 50S subunit of the bacterial ribosome.
- This binding occurs near the ribosomal exit tunnel, where the growing peptide chain emerges.

2. Inhibition of Translocation:

- The primary effect of erythromycin is to inhibit the translocation process during protein synthesis.
- Translocation is the movement of the ribosome along the messenger RNA (mRNA), allowing the ribosome to read the next codon and incorporate the appropriate amino acid into the growing polypeptide chain.
- Erythromycin prevents the movement of the ribosome along the mRNA, thereby halting the elongation of the protein chain.

3. Disruption of Peptide Chain Elongation:

- By inhibiting translocation, erythromycin disrupts the normal progression of protein synthesis.
- This disruption leads to the accumulation of incomplete polypeptide chains within the bacterial cell.

4. Bacteriostatic Effect:

- Erythromycin's interference with protein synthesis is generally bacteriostatic, meaning it inhibits bacterial growth rather than directly causing bacterial cell death.
- However, in high concentrations or against highly susceptible bacteria, erythromycin may exhibit bactericidal effects.

5. Broad Spectrum of Activity:

- Erythromycin is effective against a wide range of Gram-positive bacteria, including Streptococcus pneumoniae, Staphylococcus aureus, and Corynebacterium species.
- Some Gram-negative bacteria, such as Haemophilus influenzae and Neisseria species, are also susceptible.

6. Macrolide Class Characteristics:

- Erythromycin is part of the macrolide class of antibiotics, sharing structural and functional features with other macrolides like azithromycin and clarithromycin.

- The macrolide antibiotics are characterized by a macrocyclic lactone ring structure.

Clinical Implications:

- Erythromycin's mechanism of action makes it effective in treating various bacterial infections, especially those involving the respiratory tract, skin, and soft tissues.
- The specificity of erythromycin for bacterial ribosomes contributes to its relatively low toxicity to human cells.

Understanding the detailed mechanism of action is essential for healthcare professionals to optimize the use of erythromycin in clinical practice and minimize the risk of resistance development.

CHAPTER THREE

Indications of Erythromycin:

Erythromycin is a versatile antibiotic with a broad spectrum of activity, making it effective against various bacterial infections. The following are common indications for the use of erythromycin:

Respiratory Tract Infections:

Erythromycin is often prescribed for respiratory infections caused by susceptible organisms. This includes:
Community-acquired pneumonia.
Bronchitis.
Pertussis (whooping cough).
Legionnaires' disease.
Skin and Soft Tissue Infections:

Erythromycin is used to treat infections involving the skin and soft tissues, such as:
Cellulitis.
Erysipelas.
Impetigo.
Sexually Transmitted Infections (STIs):

Erythromycin is an alternative treatment for certain STIs, particularly when other antibiotics are not suitable. It may be used for:
Chlamydia trachomatis infections.
Syphilis in patients with penicillin allergy.
Gonorrhea in conjunction with other antibiotics.
Gastrointestinal Infections:

Erythromycin is sometimes used to treat gastrointestinal infections, including those caused by:
Campylobacter species.
Helicobacter pylori (as part of combination therapy).
Dental Infections:

Erythromycin may be prescribed for dental infections, especially in cases of penicillin allergy.
Prophylaxis in Surgery:

Erythromycin is occasionally used as a prophylactic antibiotic in certain surgical procedures to prevent postoperative infections.
Alternative in Penicillin Allergy:

Due to its different mechanism of action and structure, erythromycin is sometimes chosen as an alternative in patients with allergies to penicillin or cephalosporins.
Lyme Disease:

In some cases, erythromycin may be used for the treatment of Lyme disease, particularly when other antibiotics are not tolerated.
It's important to note that while erythromycin is effective against a range of bacteria, its use is guided by factors such as the specific pathogen involved, local resistance patterns, and individual patient characteristics. In recent years, other macrolide

antibiotics with improved pharmacokinetics and broader spectra of activity, such as azithromycin and clarithromycin, have become more commonly prescribed in certain situations. Therefore, the choice of erythromycin or alternative antibiotics depends on the clinical scenario and considerations specific to each patient.

CHAPTER FOUR

Dosage and Administration of Erythromycin:

The dosage and administration of erythromycin depend on various factors, including the specific formulation, the type and severity of the infection, patient age, weight, renal function, and individual patient characteristics. It is essential to follow the prescribing healthcare professional's recommendations and the drug manufacturer's guidelines. Below is a general overview, but specific dosing instructions should be obtained from a healthcare provider or the drug's package insert.

1. Formulations:

Erythromycin is available in various formulations, including oral tablets, capsules, oral suspensions, and intravenous (IV) formulations.

2. Oral Dosage:

Oral formulations are typically taken with or without food, depending on the specific product. However, certain formulations may be affected by food intake.

Dosages can vary, and the frequency of administration depends on the severity of the infection.

3. Intravenous (IV) Administration:

IV erythromycin is administered by healthcare professionals in a hospital setting or under close medical supervision.

The rate of IV administration is critical to prevent adverse effects, and it is usually given slowly over a specified period.

4. Pediatric Dosing:

Pediatric dosages are weight-based and age-dependent. Children may receive oral suspensions or chewable tablets to facilitate administration.

5. Dosage Adjustments:

Dosage adjustments may be necessary in patients with impaired renal function. Monitoring of drug levels and adjusting the dose accordingly is essential in these cases.

6. Compliance:

Patients should be instructed to complete the full course of erythromycin as prescribed by their healthcare provider, even if symptoms improve before completion.

7. Missed Doses:

If a dose is missed, patients should take it as soon as they remember. However, if it is almost time for the next scheduled dose, they should skip the missed dose and continue with the regular dosing schedule.

8. Drug Interactions:

Erythromycin can interact with other medications, and healthcare providers should be aware of the patient's complete medication list to avoid potential drug interactions.
Adjustments to the dosage of erythromycin or other medications may be necessary in the presence of drug interactions.
9. Monitoring:

Regular monitoring of patients receiving erythromycin is essential to assess the therapeutic response and detect any potential adverse effects.
10. Special Populations:

Special consideration is needed for pregnant or lactating women, and the risks and benefits of erythromycin use should be carefully evaluated in these populations.
It's crucial for healthcare providers to consider the patient's overall health, medical history, and potential interactions with other medications when determining the appropriate dosage and administration of erythromycin. Patients should

follow their healthcare provider's instructions and report any unusual or severe side effects promptly.

CHAPTER FIVE

Side Effects of Erythromycin:

Erythromycin is generally well-tolerated, but like any medication, it can cause side effects in some individuals. The severity and frequency of side effects can vary, and it's important for both healthcare providers and patients to be aware of potential adverse reactions. If any side effects occur, it's crucial to notify a healthcare professional promptly. Common and more serious side effects associated with erythromycin include:

1. Gastrointestinal Effects:

Nausea and Vomiting: Gastrointestinal symptoms are common, and nausea and vomiting may occur. Taking erythromycin with food can help minimize these effects.

Abdominal Pain and Cramping: Some individuals may experience abdominal discomfort or cramping.

Diarrhea: Erythromycin can disrupt the normal balance of gut bacteria, leading to diarrhea. In severe cases, this could be a sign of a more serious condition called Clostridium difficile-associated diarrhea.

2. Allergic Reactions:

Hypersensitivity Reactions: Rarely, individuals may experience allergic reactions, including rash, itching, and swelling. Severe allergic reactions, such as anaphylaxis, are extremely rare but can be life-threatening.

Stevens-Johnson Syndrome (SJS) and Toxic Epidermal Necrolysis (TEN): These are severe skin reactions that can occur rarely. They are medical emergencies and require immediate attention.

3. Liver Effects:

Hepatotoxicity: Erythromycin can cause liver enzyme elevations, and in rare cases, severe liver damage. Monitoring liver function may be necessary in certain situations.
4. Cardiovascular Effects:

QT Prolongation: Erythromycin has been associated with prolongation of the QT interval on the electrocardiogram, which can lead to a rare but serious arrhythmia known as torsades de pointes.
5. Hearing Loss (Ototoxicity):

Auditory Effects: Rare cases of hearing loss or ringing in the ears (tinnitus) have been reported with erythromycin.
6. Clostridium difficile Infection:

C. difficile-associated Diarrhea: Erythromycin, like other antibiotics, can disrupt the normal gut flora and lead to the overgrowth of Clostridium difficile bacteria, causing colitis and severe diarrhea.
7. Other Side Effects:

Pancreatitis: In rare cases, erythromycin has been associated with pancreatitis.

Visual Disturbances: Erythromycin has been reported to cause visual disturbances, including blurred vision.

Joint Pain: Some individuals may experience joint pain or inflammation.

8. Interactions with Other Medications:

Erythromycin can interact with other medications, including certain antiarrhythmics, leading to an increased risk of adverse effects.

It's important for patients to report any side effects or unusual symptoms to their healthcare provider promptly. In some cases, dosage adjustments or discontinuation of erythromycin may be necessary. Healthcare professionals should carefully consider the potential risks and benefits of erythromycin, especially in individuals with pre-existing conditions or those taking other medications.

CHAPTER SIX

Contraindications of Erythromycin:

Contraindications are specific situations or conditions in which the use of a medication like erythromycin is not recommended due to the potential risks outweighing the benefits. It's crucial for healthcare providers to carefully assess a patient's medical history and overall health to determine if erythromycin is a safe and appropriate treatment. Here are key contraindications for erythromycin:

1. Hypersensitivity to Erythromycin or Macrolide Antibiotics:

Individuals who have a known hypersensitivity or allergic reaction to erythromycin or other macrolide antibiotics (such as azithromycin or clarithromycin) should not use erythromycin.

2. Concurrent Use with Certain Medications:

Erythromycin can interact with other medications, and its use may be contraindicated when administered concurrently with drugs that have the potential for significant interactions. For example:
Terfenadine and Astemizole: Due to the risk of serious cardiac arrhythmias.
Cisapride: As it may lead to QT prolongation and arrhythmias.

3. Known QT Prolongation:

Individuals with a history of prolonged QT interval or those taking medications that can prolong the QT interval should use erythromycin with caution or avoid it altogether, as erythromycin itself has been associated with QT prolongation.

4. Pre-existing Liver Disease:

Erythromycin can affect liver function, and its use may be contraindicated in individuals with pre-existing liver disease or impaired liver function.

5. Myasthenia Gravis:

Erythromycin may exacerbate the symptoms of myasthenia gravis, a neuromuscular disorder characterized by muscle weakness and fatigue. Its use should be avoided in individuals with this condition.

6. Pregnancy and Breastfeeding:

While erythromycin is generally considered safe during pregnancy and breastfeeding, certain formulations may have limitations. It's important to discuss the risks and benefits with a healthcare provider.

7. Concomitant Use with Ergotamine and Dihydroergotamine:

Concurrent use of erythromycin with ergotamine or dihydroergotamine is contraindicated due to the potential for severe vasoconstriction and ischemia.

8. Concomitant Use with Simvastatin or Lovastatin:

Erythromycin can increase the levels of simvastatin and lovastatin, leading to an increased risk of myopathy and rhabdomyolysis. Therefore, the concurrent use of erythromycin with these statins may be contraindicated.

9. Porphyria:

Erythromycin may exacerbate symptoms of porphyria, a group of rare genetic disorders affecting the nervous system and skin.

It's important for healthcare providers to review a patient's complete medical history and current medications to identify potential contraindications before prescribing erythromycin. If contraindications are present, alternative treatment options should be considered. Always consult with a healthcare professional for personalized advice based on the individual patient's health status.

CHAPTER SEVEN

Drug Interactions with Erythromycin:

Erythromycin, like many other medications, can interact with other drugs, potentially affecting their efficacy or causing adverse effects. It's crucial for healthcare providers to be aware of potential drug interactions when prescribing erythromycin and for patients to inform their healthcare providers about all medications, supplements, and herbal products they are taking. Here are some notable drug interactions involving erythromycin:

1. Cytochrome P450 Inhibition:

Erythromycin is known to inhibit the activity of certain cytochrome P450 enzymes, particularly CYP3A4. This can affect the metabolism of other drugs that are substrates for these enzymes, leading to increased blood levels and potential toxicity. Drugs metabolized by CYP3A4 include:

Warfarin: Erythromycin can increase the anticoagulant effects of warfarin.
Theophylline: Increased theophylline levels can lead to toxicity.
Carbamazepine: Erythromycin can increase blood levels of carbamazepine.
2. QT Prolongation and Antiarrhythmics:

Erythromycin has been associated with QT prolongation, and its concurrent use with other medications that prolong the QT interval can increase the risk of serious cardiac arrhythmias. Avoid or use with caution when combined with:
Class IA and III Antiarrhythmics: (e.g., quinidine, amiodarone, sotalol)
Certain Antipsychotics: (e.g., haloperidol, thioridazine)
3. Statins:

Erythromycin can increase the levels of statins metabolized by CYP3A4, leading to an increased risk of myopathy and rhabdomyolysis. Caution is needed when erythromycin is used with statins such as:
Simvastatin

Lovastatin

4. Ergotamine and Dihydroergotamine:

Erythromycin can increase the serum levels of ergot alkaloids, leading to an increased risk of ergotism. Concomitant use is contraindicated.

5. Digoxin:

Erythromycin can increase the serum levels of digoxin, potentially leading to digoxin toxicity. Monitoring of digoxin levels is recommended during concurrent use.

6. Anticoagulants:

Erythromycin may enhance the effects of oral anticoagulants, such as warfarin, and increase the risk of bleeding. Close monitoring of prothrombin time (PT) and International Normalized Ratio (INR) is recommended.

7. Anti-HIV Medications:

Erythromycin can interact with certain antiretroviral medications used in the treatment of HIV, such as protease inhibitors and non-nucleoside reverse transcriptase inhibitors. This can affect drug levels and efficacy.

8. Calcium Channel Blockers:

Erythromycin can increase the serum levels of calcium channel blockers, leading to enhanced cardiovascular effects. Monitoring for signs of toxicity is important when using erythromycin with drugs like verapamil or diltiazem.

9. Colchicine:

Concurrent use of erythromycin with colchicine can increase the risk of colchicine toxicity, especially in individuals with renal impairment.

10. Corticosteroids:

- Erythromycin may increase the serum levels of methylprednisolone, a corticosteroid.

This list is not exhaustive, and healthcare providers should always consult drug interaction databases and consider individual patient factors when prescribing erythromycin. Patients should inform their healthcare providers about all medications they are taking, including over-the-counter drugs, supplements, and herbal products. Adjustments to dosages or alternative medications may be necessary to manage potential drug interactions.

CHAPTER EIGHT

Monitoring and Precautions for Erythromycin:

Monitoring and precautions are important aspects of ensuring the safe and effective use of erythromycin. Healthcare providers should carefully consider patient characteristics, medical history, and potential risk factors when prescribing erythromycin. Additionally, monitoring for specific parameters can help detect and manage adverse effects. Here are key aspects of monitoring and precautions associated with erythromycin:

1. Liver Function Monitoring:

Erythromycin can affect liver function, and monitoring of liver enzymes is advisable, especially in patients with pre-existing liver disease or those at risk of hepatotoxicity.

Regular liver function tests may be recommended, particularly in individuals with prolonged use of erythromycin.

2. Cardiac Monitoring:

Erythromycin has been associated with QT prolongation, and caution is advised in patients with pre-existing cardiac conditions or those taking medications that also prolong the QT interval.

Monitoring of the electrocardiogram (ECG) may be warranted in high-risk individuals.

3. Renal Function Monitoring:

Dosage adjustments may be necessary in patients with impaired renal function. Regular monitoring of renal function is advisable, especially if erythromycin is used for an extended period.

4. Monitoring for Allergic Reactions:

Patients should be monitored for signs of hypersensitivity reactions, such as rash, itching, swelling, or severe allergic reactions like anaphylaxis.

Immediate medical attention is necessary if severe allergic reactions occur.

5. Gastrointestinal Monitoring:

Monitoring for gastrointestinal side effects, such as nausea, vomiting, abdominal pain, and diarrhea, is important.
Severe or persistent diarrhea may be a sign of Clostridium difficile-associated colitis and should be promptly evaluated.

6. Monitoring Drug Levels:

Monitoring drug levels may be necessary when erythromycin is used in conjunction with medications metabolized by cytochrome P450 enzymes, as erythromycin can inhibit these enzymes and affect the metabolism of other drugs.

7. Caution in Myasthenia Gravis:

Erythromycin may exacerbate symptoms of myasthenia gravis. Close monitoring of muscle strength and function is important in individuals with this neuromuscular disorder.

8. Caution in Pregnancy and Breastfeeding:

While erythromycin is generally considered safe during pregnancy and breastfeeding, caution is warranted, and the potential risks and benefits should be discussed with healthcare providers.
9. Consideration of Patient Age and Population:

Special caution is needed in certain populations, such as the elderly and pediatric patients, as they may be more susceptible to certain adverse effects.
10. Monitoring for Drug Interactions:

Regular assessment of potential drug interactions, especially with medications metabolized by cytochrome P450 enzymes, is essential.
Adjustments to dosages or alternative medications may be necessary to manage drug interactions.
11. Patient Education and Counseling:

Patients should be educated about the importance of completing the full course of erythromycin as prescribed.
They should also be instructed to report any unusual or severe side effects promptly.
By implementing appropriate monitoring and precautions, healthcare providers can enhance the

safety and efficacy of erythromycin therapy. Individualized care, consideration of patient factors, and proactive management of potential adverse effects contribute to successful treatment outcomes.

CHAPTER NINE

Pregnancy and Lactation Considerations for Erythromycin:

Erythromycin is generally considered safe for use during pregnancy and lactation, but certain considerations should be taken into account. It's important for healthcare providers to carefully evaluate the potential risks and benefits when prescribing erythromycin to pregnant or lactating individuals.

1. Pregnancy Considerations:

Safety Profile: Erythromycin is generally considered safe for use during pregnancy. It falls into Pregnancy Category B, indicating that animal studies have not shown a risk to the fetus, but there are limited human studies.

Indications: Erythromycin may be prescribed during pregnancy to treat bacterial infections that pose a risk to the mother or fetus. Common indications include respiratory tract infections, skin and soft tissue infections, and certain sexually transmitted infections.

Gastrointestinal Motility Disorders: Erythromycin has been used to stimulate gastrointestinal motility in some cases, such as in diabetic gastroparesis. However, the benefits and risks should be carefully assessed, and alternatives may be considered.

Avoidance of Certain Formulations: While erythromycin itself is considered safe, certain formulations, such as erythromycin estolate, may be associated with an increased risk of hepatotoxicity during pregnancy. Healthcare providers may choose alternative formulations in such cases.

Monitoring: Regular monitoring and follow-up with healthcare providers are recommended to ensure the well-being of both the pregnant individual and the fetus.

2. Lactation Considerations:

Excretion in Breast Milk: Erythromycin is excreted into breast milk, but the amount is generally considered low. The decision to use erythromycin during lactation should take into account the potential benefits of treatment for the mother and the potential risks to the infant.

Infant Exposure: While exposure to erythromycin through breast milk is generally considered safe, it's important to be cautious, especially in premature or ill infants.

Breastfeeding and Newborns: Erythromycin may be used during breastfeeding, but it's advisable to monitor the infant for potential adverse effects, such as gastrointestinal disturbances or changes in bowel habits.

Alternative Antibiotics: If there are concerns about erythromycin use during breastfeeding, healthcare providers may consider alternative antibiotics with a lower risk of exposure through breast milk.

Communication with Healthcare Provider: Open communication between the healthcare provider and the breastfeeding individual is crucial. It allows for informed decision-making and ongoing monitoring of the infant's well-being.

Overall Recommendations:

Erythromycin can be used during pregnancy and lactation when the potential benefits outweigh the potential risks.
Healthcare providers should carefully evaluate the specific circumstances, considering the indication for treatment and the available alternatives.
Open communication and collaboration between the patient and healthcare provider are essential to make informed decisions regarding the use of erythromycin during pregnancy and lactation.
It's important for pregnant or breastfeeding individuals to discuss their medical history, current health status, and any concerns with their healthcare providers before starting or continuing erythromycin therapy. This allows for personalized decision-making and optimal management of

bacterial infections while minimizing potential risks to the mother and infant.

CHAPTER TEN

Overdose and Emergency Management of Erythromycin:

Overdose with erythromycin can lead to an increased risk of adverse effects, including gastrointestinal symptoms and cardiac complications. Emergency management focuses on supportive care, minimizing absorption, and addressing specific symptoms. It's important for individuals who suspect an overdose or experience severe symptoms to seek immediate medical attention. Here are considerations for the overdose and emergency management of erythromycin:

1. Symptoms of Overdose:

Overdose symptoms may include severe nausea, vomiting, abdominal pain, diarrhea, and potentially

serious cardiac effects such as arrhythmias (including QT prolongation).
2. Seek Medical Attention:

In case of suspected overdose, individuals should seek immediate medical attention by calling emergency services or going to the nearest emergency room.
3. Emergency Management:

Supportive Care: The primary approach to erythromycin overdose involves supportive care. This includes monitoring and treating symptoms such as nausea, vomiting, and abdominal pain. Intravenous fluids may be administered to maintain hydration.

Activated Charcoal: Administration of activated charcoal may be considered to help reduce further absorption of erythromycin, especially if presented shortly after ingestion. However, its effectiveness decreases with time after ingestion.

Gastric Lavage: In some cases, gastric lavage (stomach pumping) may be considered, particularly if the ingestion occurred within a short time frame. This procedure is generally reserved for severe cases and is performed under medical supervision.

Monitoring Electrolytes and ECG: Due to the potential for QT prolongation and cardiac arrhythmias, continuous monitoring of the electrocardiogram (ECG) and periodic assessment of electrolyte levels (especially potassium and magnesium) may be necessary.

Management of Severe Symptoms: Severe symptoms may require additional interventions. For example, if there are signs of arrhythmias, specific antiarrhythmic medications or electrical cardioversion may be considered under medical supervision.

4. Specific Antidote:

There is no specific antidote for erythromycin overdose. Management is largely supportive, addressing symptoms and preventing further absorption.

5. Consultation with Poison Control Center:

Healthcare providers may consult with a regional poison control center for guidance on managing erythromycin overdose. Poison control centers can provide expertise and advice on specific cases.
6. Discontinuation of Erythromycin:

In cases of overdose, the healthcare provider may decide to discontinue erythromycin treatment. The decision will depend on the severity of the overdose, the presence of symptoms, and the patient's overall health status.
7. Follow-up:

Individuals who have experienced an overdose should follow up with their healthcare provider for ongoing monitoring and assessment. Long-term complications are rare but may occur, especially if severe cardiac effects were present.
It's important to note that the information provided here is general, and actual emergency management may vary based on the individual case and specific circumstances. Immediate medical attention and consultation with healthcare

professionals are crucial in cases of suspected overdose.

CHAPTER ELEVEN

Patient Counseling for Erythromycin:

Effective patient counseling is essential to ensure that individuals prescribed erythromycin understand how to take the medication, are aware of potential side effects, and can actively participate in their treatment plan. Here's a comprehensive guide to patient counseling for erythromycin:

1. Medication Information:

Name and Purpose: Explain the name of the medication (erythromycin) and its purpose as an antibiotic used to treat bacterial infections.

Formulation: Discuss the specific formulation prescribed (tablet, capsule, suspension, or intravenous) and the importance of taking the correct form as directed.

2. Dosage and Administration:

Dosage Instructions: Clearly explain the prescribed dosage, including the number of tablets or capsules and the frequency of administration.

Timing of Administration: Provide instructions on whether erythromycin should be taken with or without food and the importance of adhering to the recommended schedule.

Completion of Course: Emphasize the importance of completing the entire course of medication, even if symptoms improve before the medication is finished.

3. Potential Side Effects:

Common Side Effects: Discuss potential common side effects, such as nausea, vomiting, abdominal pain, and diarrhea, and reassure the patient that these symptoms are generally temporary.

Allergic Reactions: Highlight signs of allergic reactions, including rash, itching, swelling, and difficulty breathing, and instruct the patient to seek immediate medical attention if any of these occur.

Gastrointestinal Effects: Provide guidance on managing gastrointestinal symptoms, such as taking erythromycin with food to reduce the risk of stomach upset.

4. Drug Interactions:

Other Medications: Instruct patients to inform healthcare providers about all medications, including over-the-counter drugs, supplements, and herbal products, to avoid potential drug interactions. Specific Medications to Avoid: Highlight specific medications (e.g., certain antiarrhythmics, statins) that may interact with erythromycin, and advise patients to consult their healthcare provider before starting new medications.

5. Pregnancy and Lactation Considerations:

Communication with Healthcare Provider: Encourage pregnant or breastfeeding individuals to discuss their situation with their healthcare provider to assess the risks and benefits of erythromycin use.

Monitoring: Emphasise the importance of regular monitoring and follow-up appointments during pregnancy or lactation.

6. Missed Doses:

Instructions for Missed Doses: Advise patients on what to do if they miss a dose, instructing them to take the missed dose as soon as they remember or skip it if it's almost time for the next scheduled dose.

7. Precautions:

Driving and Operating Machinery: Caution patients about potential dizziness or lightheadedness associated with erythromycin and advise against driving or operating heavy machinery if these symptoms occur.

Avoiding Alcohol: Recommend avoiding excessive alcohol consumption while taking erythromycin, as it may enhance the risk of certain side effects.

8. Follow-Up and Reporting:

Scheduled Follow-up: Schedule follow-up appointments to monitor progress and address any concerns or side effects.

Reporting Unusual Symptoms: Instruct patients to report any unusual or severe symptoms to their healthcare provider promptly.

9. Storage and Expiry:

Proper Storage: Advise on proper storage conditions for erythromycin, including temperature requirements and protection from light.
Expiry Date: Emphasise the importance of not using expired medication and proper disposal of any unused medication.
10. General Health Tips:

Hydration: Encourage patients to stay well-hydrated, especially if experiencing gastrointestinal symptoms.
Sun Protection: If photosensitivity is a known side effect, advise patients to use sun protection measures.
11. Questions and Concerns:

Open Communication: Encourage patients to ask questions and express any concerns they may have about the medication.
Contact Information: Provide contact information for the healthcare provider or pharmacy in case of questions or emergencies.

Effective patient counselling fosters understanding, adherence, and a collaborative approach to healthcare. Tailor the counselling to the individual patient's needs and ensure that they feel comfortable and informed about their treatment with erythromycin.